The Complete Dash Diet Main & Side Dish Cookbook

Easy Dash Diet Main & Side Dish Recipes For Everyone

Peter Haley

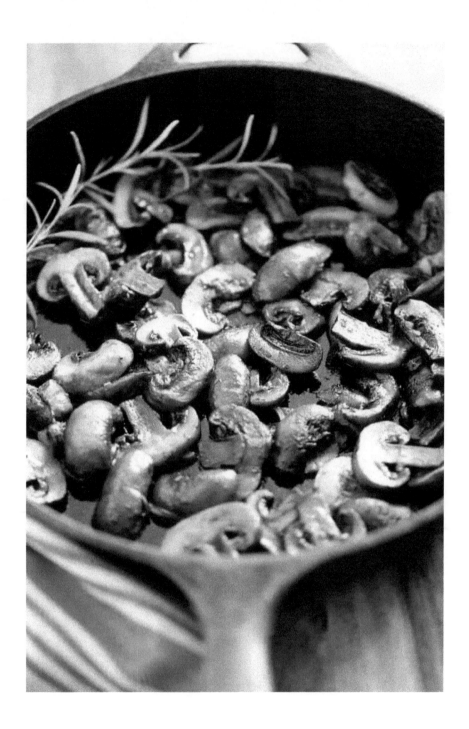

Table of contents

Asparagus with Lemon Sauce

Prep Time: 5 mins

Servings: 4

Cooking: 15 mins

Ingredients:

- 20 medium asparagus spears, rinsed and trimmed
- 1 fresh lemon, rinsed (for peel and juice)
- 2 tbsps reduced-fat mayonnaise
- 1 tbsp dried parsley
- 1/8 tsp ground black pepper

Directions:

1. Place 1 inch of water in a 4-quart pot with a lid. Place a steamer basket inside the pot, and add asparagus.
2. Cover and bring to a boil over high heat. Reduce heat to medium. Cook for 5–10 mins, until asparagus is easily pierced with a sharp knife. Do not overcook.

3. While the asparagus cooks, grate the lemon zest into a small bowl. Cut the lemon in half and squeeze the juice into the bowl. Use the back of a spoon to press out extra juice and remove pits. Add mayonnaise, parsley, pepper, and salt. Stir well. Set aside.

4. When the asparagus is tender, remove the pot from the heat. Place asparagus spears in a serving bowl. Drizzle the lemon sauce evenly over the asparagus (about 1-1/2 tsps per portion) and serve.

Nutrition:

- Calories 39
- Fat 0 g

Autumn Salad

Prep Time: 5 mins

Servings: 6

Ingredients:

- 1 medium Granny Smith apple, sliced thinly (with skin)
- 2 tbsps lemon juice
- 1 bag (about 5 cups) mixed lettuce greens (or your favorite lettuce)
- 1/2 cup dried cranberries n 1/4 cup walnuts, chopped
- 1/4 cup unsalted sunflower seeds
- 1/3 cup low-fat raspberry vinaigrette dressing

Directions:

1. Sprinkle lemon juice on the apple slices.
2. Mix the lettuce, cranberries, apple, walnuts, and sunflower seeds in a bowl.
3. Toss with 1/3 cup of raspberry vinaigrette dressing, to lightly cover the salad.

Nutrition:

- Calories 138
- Fat 7 g
- Protein 3 g
- Carbs 19 g

Broccoli and Cheese

Prep Time: 5 mins

Servings: 4

Cooking: 15 mins

Ingredients:

- 6 cups fresh broccoli, rinsed and cut into bite-sized florets (or substitute 6 cups frozen broccoli, thawed and warmed, and skip step 1)

For sauce

- 1 cup fat-free evaporated milk
- 1 tbsp cornstarch
- 1/2 cup shredded cheddar cheese
- 1/4 tsp Worcestershire sauce
- 1/4 tsp hot sauce
- 1 slice whole-wheat bread, diced and toasted (for croutons)

Directions:

1. Bring a large pot of water to boil over high heat. Add fresh broccoli, and cook until easily pierced by a fork, about 7–10 mins. Drain and set aside.
2. In a separate saucepan, combine evaporated milk and cornstarch. Slowly bring to a boil while stirring often.
3. When the milk comes to a boil, remove it from the heat and add the cheese. Continue to stir until the cheese is melted and evenly mixed.
4. Add the Worcestershire and hot sauces, and stir.
5. Pour cheese over hot broccoli.
6. Sprinkle whole-wheat croutons over broccoli and cheese mixture, and serve.

Nutrition:

- Calories 162
- Fat 5 g
- Fiber 4 g
- Protein 11 g
- Carbs 19 g

Caribbean Casserole

Prep Time: 5 mins

Servings: 10

Cooking: 10 mins

Ingredients:

- 1 medium onion, chopped
- 1/2 green pepper, diced
- 1 tbsp canola oil
- 1 14-1/2-ounce can stewed tomatoes
- 1 16-ounce can black beans (or beans of your choice)
- 1 tsp oregano leaves
- 1/2 tsp garlic powder
- 1-1/2 cups instant brown rice, uncooked

Directions:

1. Sauté onion and green pepper in canola oil, in a large pan, until tender. Do not brown.

2. Add tomatoes, beans (include liquid from both), oregano, and garlic powder. Bring to a boil. Stir in rice and cover. Reduce heat to simmer for 5 mins. Remove from heat and let stand for 5 mins.

Nutrition:

- Calories 185
- Fat 1 g
- Protein 7 g
- Carbs 37 g

Avocado Garden Salad

Prep Time: 5 mins

Servings: 6

Cooking: 10 mins

Ingredients:

- 6 cups torn or cut mixed salad greens
- 3 medium tomatoes, chopped
- 5 green onions, chopped
- 1 small cucumber, peeled and chopped
- 2 tbsps lemon juice
- 1/3 tsp garlic powder
- 1/2 tsp ground black pepper
- 1/2 tsp salt
- 1 large avocado, peeled

Directions:

Combine all the ingredients and serve.

Nutrition:

- Calories 78
- Carbs 9 g
- Fiber 4 g
- Protein 2 g
- Fat 5 g

Oven-Fried Yucca

Prep Time: 5 mins

Servings: 6

Cooking: 35 mins

Ingredients:

- 1 lb fresh yucca (cassava), cut into 3-inch sections and peeled (or 1 lb peeled frozen yucca)
- nonstick cooking oil spray

Directions:

1. In a kettle, combine the yucca with enough cold water to cover it by 1 inch. Bring the water to a boil, and slowly simmer the yucca for 20 to 30 mins, or until it is tender.
2. Preheat oven to 350° F.
3. Transfer the yucca with a slotted spoon to a cutting board, let it cool, and cut it lengthwise into 3/4-inch-wide wedges, discarding the thin woody core.

4. Spray cookie sheet with the nonstick cooking oil spray. Spread yucca wedges on cookie sheet, and spray wedges with cooking oil spray. Cover with foil paper and bake for 8 mins. Uncover and return to oven to bake for an additional 7 mins.

Nutrition:

- Calories 91
- Fat 1 g
- Fiber 4 g
- Protein 11 g
- Carbs 19 g

Celery with Cheese Mousse

Prep Time: 5 mins

Servings: 4

Ingredients:

- 1/4 cup low-fat whipped cream cheese
- 1/4 cup fat-free plain yogurt
- 2 tbsps scallions (green onions), rinsed and chopped
- 1 tbsp lemon juice
- 1/2 tsp ground black pepper
- 6 celery sticks, rinsed, with ends cut off
- 1 tbsp chopped walnuts

Directions:

1. Combine cream cheese, yogurt, scallions, lemon juice, and pepper. Mix well with a wooden spoon.
2. Spread mixture evenly down the middle of each celery stick.
3. Cut each stick into 5 pieces. Top with chopped walnuts, and serve.

Nutrition:

- Calories 35
- Fiber 1 g
- Protein 2 g
- Carbs 3 g
- Fat 2 g

Chicken Tomatillo Salad

Prep Time: 5 mins

Servings: 6

Cooking: 20 mins

Ingredients:

Dressing

- 1 cup husked and quartered tomatillos
- 3 tbsp light Italian dressing
- 1 fresh Anaheim chili, seeded and chopped
- 1/4 tsp ground black pepper

Salad

- 2 cups chopped, cooked chicken or turkey
- 1 cup chopped red bell pepper
- 1 cup frozen corn, thawed
- 1 cup chopped carrots
- 4 green onions, sliced
- 1/4 cup chopped fresh cilantro

Directions:

1. In a blender or food processor container, purée tomatillos with dressing, Anaheim chili, and ground black pepper; set aside.
2. Combine all salad ingredients: in a large bowl and toss.
3. Drizzle dressing over salad and toss well to coat.
4. Cover and chill for 20 mins or make a day ahead to allow flavors to blend.
5. Serve on lettuce-lined plates or bowls.

Nutrition:

- Calories 141
- Carbs 12 g
- Protein 16 g
- Fat 4 g

Green Beans Sauté

Prep Time: 5 mins

Servings: 6

Cooking: 20 mins

Ingredients:

- 1 lb fresh or frozen green beans, cut in 1-inch pieces
- 1 tbsp vegetable oil
- 1 large yellow onion, halved lengthwise and thinly sliced
- 1 tbsp fresh parsley, minced

Directions:

1. If using fresh green beans, cook green beans in boiling water for 10-12 mins or steam for 2-3 mins until barely fork tender. Drain well. If using frozen green beans, thaw first.
2. Heat oil in a large skillet. Sauté onion until golden.
3. Stir in green beans, salt and pepper. Heat through.

4. Toss with parsley before serving.

Nutrition:

- Calories 64
- Fiber 1 g
- Protein 2 g
- Carbs 3 g
- Fat 2 g

Romaine Lettuce With Dressing

Prep Time: 5 mins

Servings: 4

Ingredients:

- 1 slice whole wheat-bread
- 2 heads romaine lettuce, rinsed and halved lengthwise
- 4 tsp olive oil
- 4 tsp light Caesar dressing
- 4 tbsp shredded parmesan cheese
- 16 cherry tomatoes, rinsed and halved

Directions:

1. Preheat grill pan on high temperature.
2. Cube the bread. Spread in a single layer on a foil-covered tray for a toaster oven or conventional oven. Toast to a medium-brown color and crunchy texture. Remove. Allow to cool.
3. Brush the cut side of each half of romaine lettuce with 1 tsp of olive oil.

4. Place cut side down on a grill pan on the stovetop. Cook just until grill marks appear and romaine is heated through, about 2–5 mins.

5. Place each romaine half on a large salad plate. Top each with one-fourth of the bread cubes. Drizzle each with 1 tsp of light Caesar dressing. Sprinkle each with 1 tbsp of shredded parmesan cheese. Garnish with eight tomato halves around each plate.

Nutrition:

- Calories 162
- Carbohydrate 17 g
- Dietary Fiber 2 g
- Protein 1 g
- Total Fat 1

Corn and Green Chili Salad

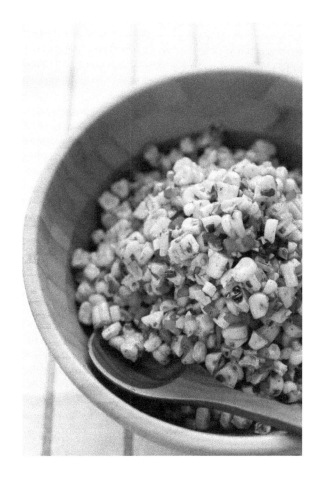

Prep Time: 5 mins

Servings: 4

Ingredients:

- 2 cups frozen corn, thawed
- 1 (10-ounce) can diced tomatoes with green chilies, drained
- 1/2 tbsp vegetable oil
- 1 tbsp lime juice
- 1/3 cup sliced green onions
- 2 tbsps chopped fresh cilantro

Directions:

Combine all Ingredients in a medium bowl; mix well and serve.

Nutrition:

- Calories 94
- Carbs 19 g
- Protein 3 g
- Fat 2 g

Avocado appetizer

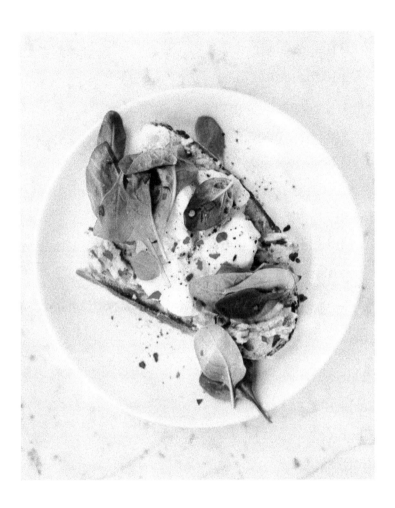

Prep Time: 7 mins

Servings: 4

Ingredients:

- 1 tbsp vinegar
- 2 tbsp moustard
- 2 tbsps lemon juice
- 1/3 tsp garlic powder
- 1/2 tsp ground black pepper
- 2 large avocado, divided in two parts

Directions:

Combine all the ingredients and put the vinaigrette on top of each half avocado and serve.

Nutrition:

- Calories 78
- Carbs 8 g
- Fiber 5 g
- Protein 4 g
- Fat 5 g

Cabbage and Tomato Salad

Prep Time: 5 mins

Servings: 8

Ingredients:

- 1 small head cabbage, sliced thinly
- 2 medium tomatoes, cut in cubes
- 1 cup sliced radishes
- 2 tsps olive oil
- 2 tbsp rice vinegar (or lemon juice)
- 2 tbsp fresh cilantro, chopped

Directions:

1. In a large bowl, mix together the cabbage, tomatoes, and radishes.
2. In another bowl, mix together the rest of the ingredients and pour over the vegetables.

Nutrition:

- Calories 41
- Carbohydrate 7 g
- Dietary Fiber 2 g
- Protein 1 g
- Total Fat 1

Creole Green Beans

Prep Time: 5 mins

Servings: 8

Cooking: 7 mins

Ingredients:

- 2 tsp vegetable oil
- 2 small cloves garlic, chopped
- 1 (16-ounce) package frozen cut green beans
- 1 cup chopped red bell pepper
- 1 cup chopped fresh tomatoes
- 1/2 cup chopped celery
- 1/4 tsp cayenne pepper

Directions:

1. Heat oil in a large skillet over low heat.
2. Sauté garlic in oil for 1 minute.
3. Add green beans and bell peppers; increase heat to medium and cook for 7 mins.

4. Stir in tomatoes, celery, and seasonings; cook for 7 mins more. Serve while hot.

Nutrition:

- Calories 35
- Carbohydrate 6 g
- Fiber 2 g
- Protein 1 g
- Total Fat 1 g

Mango and Blackeye Pea Salsa

Prep Time: 5 mins

Servings: 10

Ingredients:

- 1 (15-1/2-ounce) can black-eyed peas, drained and rinsed
- 1-1/2 tomatoes, finely chopped
- 1 mango, peeled and finely chopped
- 2 green onions, chopped
- 1 tbsp vegetable oil
- 1 tbsp white vinegar
- juice of half a lime
- 1 tsp ground cumin
- 1/2 tsp garlic powder

Directions:

1. In a large bowl, combine all ingredients and mix well.
2. Serve immediately or cover and refrigerate for up to 4 hours to allow the flavors to blend.
3. Serve with baked pita or corn chips.

Nutrition:

- Calories 83
- Carbohydrate 14 g
- Fiber 2 g
- Protein 1 g
- Total Fat 1

Garden Potato Salad

Prep Time: 10 mins

Servings: 10

Ingredients:

- 3 lbs (about 6 large) potatoes, boiled in jackets, peeled and cut into 1/2-inch cubes
- 1 cup chopped celery
- 1/2 cup sliced green onion
- 2 tbsps chopped parsley
- 1 cup low-fat cottage cheese
- 3/4 cup skim milk
- 3 tbsp lemon juice
- 2 tbsp cider vinegar
- 1/2 tsp celery seed
- 1/2 tsp dill weed
- 1/2 tsp dry mustard

Directions:

1. In a large bowl, place potatoes, celery, green onion, and parsley.

2. Meanwhile, in a blender or food processor, blend cottage cheese, milk, lemon juice, vinegar, celery seed, dill weed, dry mustard, and white pepper until smooth. Chill for 1 hour.
3. Pour chilled cottage cheese mixture over vegetables; mix well. Chill at least 30 mins before serving.

Nutrition:

- Calories 151
- Carbs 11 g
- Fiber 6 g
- Protein 3 g
- Total Fat 1 g

Oven Fries

Prep Time: 10 mins

Servings: 4

Cooking: 14 mins

Ingredients:

- nonstick cooking spray
- 2 large russet potatoes, cut into wedges

Seasoning Mix

- 2 cloves garlic, finely chopped
- 1 tsp Italian herb seasoning mix
- 1 tsp chili powder and/or paprika

Directions:

1. Preheat oven to 400°F.
2. Spray a cookie sheet with nonstick cooking spray. Place potato wedges on the cookie sheet.

3. In a small bowl, combine garlic with seasonings and sprinkle 1/2 of the mixture over the top of the potato wedges.

4. Bake wedges for about 7 mins or until they start to brown. Flip wedges over. Sprinkle with the remaining mixture, and bake for another 7 mins or until the wedges are browned and cooked through. Serve while hot.

Nutrition:

- Calories 146
- Carbs 33 g
- Fiber 6 g
- Protein 3 g
- Fat 8 g

Parmesan Rice and Pasta

Prep Time: 10 mins

Servings: 4

Cooking: 25 mins

Ingredients:

- 2 tbsp olive oil
- 1/2 cup finely broken vermicelli, uncooked
- 2 tbsp diced onion
- 1 cup long-grain white rice, uncooked
- 1-1/4 cups hot chicken stock
- 1-1/4 cups hot water
- 1 bay leaf
- 2 tbsp grated parmesan cheese

Directions:

1. In a large skillet, heat oil. Sauté vermicelli and onion until golden brown, about 2 to 4 mins over medium-high heat. Drain off oil.

2. Add rice, stock, water, pepper, and bay leaf. Cover and simmer 15-20 mins. Fluff with fork. Cover and let stand 5-20 mins. Remove bay leaf.
3. Sprinkle with cheese and serve immediately.

Nutrition:

- Calories 172
- Carbs 11 g
- Fiber 6 g
- Protein 3 g
- Total Fat 1 g

Potato Sauté with Onions

Prep Time: 10 mins

Servings: 4

Cooking: 15 mins

Ingredients:

- 2 cups water
- 2 large russet potatoes, cleaned and cut in half
- 1 tbsp vegetable oil
- 1/2 cup chopped onion
- 1/2 cup no salt added canned corn or frozen corn, thawed
- 1/2 cup chopped tomato
- 1/2 tsp oregano
- 1/4 cup crumbled reduced fat Monterey Jack cheese

Directions:

1. Bring water to a boil in a large pan. Add potatoes and cook until crisp-tender, about 15 mins. Drain well and cut into bite-size pieces.
2. Heat oil in a large skillet. Sauté onion until golden brown and soft. Add potatoes and cook over medium-high heat, stirring frequently, until golden brown.
3. Stir in corn, tomato, oregano, salt, and ground black pepper. Top with cheese and serve.

Nutrition:

- Calories 217
- Carbs 39 g
- Fiber 6 g
- Protein 6 g
- Fat 5 g

Garlic Mashed Potatoes

Prep Time: 10 mins

Servings: 4

Cooking: 45 mins

Ingredients:

- 1 lb (about 2 large) potatoes, peeled and quartered
- 2 cups skim milk
- 2 large cloves garlic, chopped
- 1/2 tsp white pepper

Directions:

1. Cook potatoes, covered, in a small amount of boiling water for 20-25 mins or until tender. Remove from heat. Drain and recover.
2. Meanwhile, in a small saucepan over low heat, cook garlic in milk until garlic is soft, about 30 mins.

3. Add milk-garlic mixture and white pepper to potatoes. Beat with an electric mixer on low speed or mash with a potato masher until smooth.

<u>Microwave Directions</u>

4. Scrub potatoes, pat dry, and prick with a fork. On a plate, cook potatoes, uncovered, on 100% power (high) until tender, about 12 mins, turning potatoes over once. Let stand 5 mins. Peel and quarter. Meanwhile, in a 4-cup glass measuring cup, combine milk and garlic. Cook, uncovered, on 50% power (medium) until garlic is soft, about 4 mins. Continue as directed above.

Nutrition:

- Calories 141
- Carbohydrate 18 g
- Fiber 2 g
- Protein 1 g
- Total Fat 1 g

Red Hot Fusilli

Prep Time: 10 mins

Servings: 4

Cooking: 15 mins

Ingredients:

- 1 tbsp olive oil
- 2 cloves garlic, minced
- 1/4 cup freshly minced parsley
- 4 cups ripe tomatoes, chopped
- 1 tbsp fresh basil, chopped or 1 tsp dried basil
- 1 tbsp oregano leaves, crushed or 1 tsp dried oregano
- ground red pepper or cayenne to taste
- 8 oz uncooked fusilli pasta (4 cups cooked)

Directions:

1. Heat oil in a medium saucepan. Sauté garlic and parsley until golden.

2. Add tomatoes and spices. Cook uncovered over low heat 15 mins or until thickened, stirring frequently.
3. Cook pasta firm in unsalted water.
4. To serve, spoon sauce over pasta and sprinkle with coarsely chopped parsley

Nutrition:

- Calories 304
- Carbs 39 g
- Fiber 6 g
- Protein 6 g
- Fat 5 g

Egg and Beans

Prep Time: 5 mins

Servings: 3

Ingredients:

- 5 beaten eggs
- 1 tsp. chili powder
- 2 chopped garlic cloves
- ½ cup milk
- ½ cup tomato sauce
- 1 cup cooked white beans

Directions:

1. Add milk and eggs to a bowl and mix well
2. Add the rest of the ingredients: and mix well
3. Add a cup of water to the pot
4. Transfer the bowl to your pot and lock up the lid
5. Cook on HIGH pressure for 18 mins
6. Release the pressure naturally over 10 mins
7. Serve with warm bread

Nutrition:

- Calories 206
- Fat 9 g
- Carbs 23 g
- Protein 9 g

Glazed Carrots

Prep Time: 5 mins

Servings: 4

Cooking: 10 mins

Ingredients:

- 4 cups baby carrots, rinsed and split lengthwise if very thick (or frozen pre-sliced carrots)
- 2 tbsps soft tub margarine
- 2 tbsps brown sugar
- 1/2 tsp ground cinnamon

Directions:

1. Place the carrots in a small saucepan. Add just enough water to barely cover the carrots. Cover. Bring to a boil. Cook for 7–8 mins
2. Combine margarine, brown sugar, cinnamon, and salt in a small saucepan, and melt together over low heat (or put in a microwave-safe bowl and microwave for a

few seconds on high power, until margarine is mostly melted). Stir well to combine ingredients.

3. Drain carrots, leaving them in the saucepan. Pour cinnamon mixture over carrots. Cook and stir over medium heat for 2–3 mins, just until carrots are thoroughly coated and the glaze thickens slightly

Nutrition:

- Calories 67
- Fat 3 g
- Fiber 2 g
- Protein 1 g
- Carbs 10 g

Fresh Cabbage and Tomato Salad

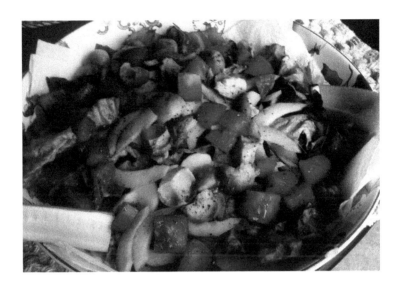

Prep Time: 5 mins

Servings: 8

Ingredients:

- 1 small head cabbage, sliced thinly
- 2 medium tomatoes, cut in cubes
- 1 cup sliced radishes
- 2 tsps olive oil
- 2 tbsps rice vinegar (or lemon juice)

- 1/2 tsp red pepper
- 2 tbsps fresh cilantro, chopped

Directions:

1. In a large bowl, mix together the cabbage, tomatoes, and radishes.
2. In another bowl, mix together the rest of the ingredients: and pour over the vegetables.

Nutrition:

- Calories 41
- Fat 1 g

Garlic Mashed Potatoes

Prep Time: 5 mins

Servings: 4

Cooking: 35 mins

Ingredients:

- 1 lb (about 2 large) potatoes, peeled and quartered
- 2 cups skim milk
- 2 large cloves garlic, chopped

Directions:

1. Cook potatoes, covered, in a small amount of boiling water for 20-25 mins or until tender. Remove from heat. Drain and recover.
2. Meanwhile, in a small saucepan over low heat, cook garlic in milk until garlic is soft, about 30 mins.
3. Add milk-garlic mixture and white pepper to potatoes. Beat with an electric mixer on low speed or mash with a potato masher until smooth.

55

4. Scrub potatoes, pat dry, and prick with a fork. On a plate, cook potatoes, uncovered, on 100% power (high) until tender, about 12 mins, turning potatoes over once. Let stand 5 mins. Peel and quarter. Meanwhile, in a 4-cup glass measuring cup, combine milk and garlicup Cook, uncovered, on 50% power (medium) until garlic is soft, about 4 mins. Continue as directed above.

Nutrition:

- Calories 141
- Fat less than 1 g

Cheddar and Apple Sandwich

Prep Time: 5 mins

Servings: 2

Ingredients:

- Cooking spray
- ½ cup arugula
- 4 whole-wheat bread slices
- 4 low-fat cheddar cheese slices
- 2 tbsp low-fat honey mustard
- 1 thinly sliced apple

Directions:

1. Set Panini press on medium heat.
2. Spread the mustard on each slice of the bread. Lay the apple on two of the bread slices, top with cheese and then the arugula. Top with the other two slices of bread.
3. Coat the Panini press with cooking spray and grill each sandwich for 4-5 mins.
4. Allow to cool before serving.

Nutrition:

- Calories 22
- Fat 4 g
- Carbs 23 g
- Protein 11 g

Herbed Potato Salad

Prep Time: 5 mins

Servings: 6

Cooking: 10 mins

Ingredients:

- 1-1/2 lbs red potatoes (about 8 potatoes), cut into cubes
- 1/2 cup light Italian dressing
- 1/2 tbsp spicy brown mustard
- 1 tbsp chopped fresh parsley
- 1 tsp garlic salt
- 1/4 tsp ground black pepper
- 1/2 cup chopped red bell pepper
- 1/2 cup chopped green bell pepper
- 1/2 cup chopped green onions

Directions:

1. In a large pot, cook potatoes in boiling water until tender, about 10 mins (do not overcook).
2. Drain well and let cool.
3. Cut potatoes into bite-size pieces and place in a medium bowl.
4. In a small bowl, combine dressing, mustard, parsley, and seasonings; pour over potatoes and toss well.
5. Carefully stir in bell peppers and green onions. Cover and chill until ready to serve.

Nutrition:

- Calories 132
- Carbs 24 g
- Fiber 4 g
- Protein 2 g
- Fat 4 g

Herbed Vegetable Mix

Prep Time: 5 mins

Servings: 7

Cooking: 13 mins

Ingredients:

- 2 tbsps water
- 1 cup thinly sliced zucchini
- 1-1/4 cups thinly sliced yellow squash
- 1/2 cup green bell pepper, cut into 2-inch strips
- 1/4 cup celery, cut into 2-inch strips
- 1/4 cup chopped onion
- 1/2 tsp caraway seeds
- 1/8 tsp garlic powder
- 1 medium tomato, cut into 8 wedges

Directions:

1. Heat water in a medium pan. Add zucchini, squash, bell pepper, celery, and onion.

2. Cover and cook over medium heat until vegetables are crisp-tender, about 4 mins.
3. Sprinkle seasonings over vegetables. Top with tomato wedges.
4. Cover again and cook over low heat until tomato wedges are warm, about 2 mins. Serve warm.

Nutrition:

- Calories 24
- Carbs 5 g
- Fiber 4 g
- Protein 2 g
- Fat 4 g

Limas and Spinach

Prep Time: 5 mins

Servings: 7

Cooking: 13 mins

Ingredients:

- 2 cups frozen lima beans
- 1 tbsp vegetable oil
- 1 cup fennel, cut in 4-inch strips
- 1/2 cup onion, chopped
- 1/4 cup low-sodium chicken broth
- 4 cups leaf spinach, washed thoroughly
- 1 tbsp distilled vinegar
- 1/8 tsp black pepper
- 1 tbsp raw chives

Directions:

1. Steam or boil lima beans in unsalted water for about 10 mins. Drain.

63

2. In skillet, sauté onions and fennel in oil.

3. Add beans and broth to onions and cover. Cook for 2 mins.

4. Stir in spinach. Cover and cook until spinach has wilted, about 2 mins.

5. Stir in vinegar and pepper. Cover and let stand for 30 seconds.

6. Sprinkle with chives and serve.

Nutrition:

- Calories 93
- Fat 2 g
- Protein 5 g
- Carbs 15 g

Easy Chickpea Veggie Burgers

Prep Time: 10 mins

Servings: 4

Cooking: 20 mins

Ingredients:

- 1 15-ounce can chickpeas, drained and rinsed
- ½ cup frozen spinach, thawed
- ⅓ cup rolled oats
- 1 tsp garlic powder
- 1 tsp onion powder

Directions:

1. Preheat oven to 400°F. Grease a sheet or line one with parchment paper and set aside.
2. In a mixing bowl, add half of the beans and mash with a fork until fairly smooth. Set aside.
3. Add the remaining half of the beans, spinach, oats, and spices to a food processor or blender and blend until

65

puréed. Add the mixture to the bowl of mashed beans and stir until well combined.

4. Divide mixture into 4 equal portions and shape into patties. Bake for 7 to 10 mins. Carefully turn over and bake for another 7 to 10 mins or until crusty on the outside.

5. Place on a whole grain bun with your favorite toppings.

Nutrition:

- Calories 118
- Fat 1g
- Carbs 21g
- Fiber 7g
- Protein 7g

Cinnamon-Scented Quinoa

Prep Time: 5 mins

Servings: 4

Ingredients:

- Chopped walnuts
- 1 ½ cup water
- Maple syrup
- 2 cinnamon sticks
- 1 cup quinoa

Directions:

1. Add the quinoa to a bowl and wash it in several changes of water until the water is clear. When washing quinoa, rub grains and allow them to settle before you pour off the water.

2. Use a large fine-mesh sieve to drain the quinoa. Prepare your pressure cooker with a trivet and steaming basket. Place the quinoa and the cinnamon sticks in the basket and pour the water.

3. Close and lock the lid. Cook at high pressure for 6 mins. When the cooking time is up, release the pressure using the quick release method.
4. Fluff the quinoa with a fork and remove the cinnamon sticks. Divide the cooked quinoa among serving bowls and top with maple syrup and chopped walnuts.

Nutrition:

- Calories 160
- Fat 3 g
- Carbs 28 g
- Protein 6 g

Thyme Mushrooms

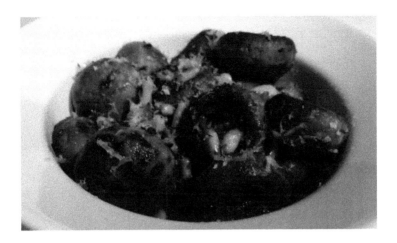

Prep Time: 10 mins

Servings: 4

Ingredients:

- 1 tbsp chopped thyme
- 2 tbsp olive oil
- 2 tbsp chopped parsley
- 4 minced garlic cloves
- Black pepper
- 2 lbs. halved white mushrooms

Directions:

1. In a baking pan, combine the mushrooms with the garlic and the other Ingredients, toss, introduce in the oven and cook at 400 º F for 30 mins.
2. Divide between plates and serve.

Nutrition:

- Calories 251
- Fat 9.3 g
- Carbs 13.2 g
- Protein 6 g

Rosemary Endives

Prep Time: 10 mins

Servings: 4

Ingredients:

- 2 tbsp olive oil
- 1 tsp. dried rosemary
- 2 halved endives
- ¼ tsp. black pepper
- ½ tsp. turmeric powder

Directions:

1. In a baking pan, combine the endives with the oil and the other ingredients, toss gently, introduce in the oven and bake at 400 º F for 20 mins.
2. Divide between plates and serve.

Nutrition:

- Calories 66
- Fat 7.1 g
- Carbs 1.2 g
- Protein 0.3 g

Roasted Beets

Prep Time: 10 mins

Servings: 4

Ingredients:

- 2 minced garlic cloves
- ¼ tsp. black pepper
- 4 peeled and sliced beets
- ¼ cup chopped walnuts
- 2 tbsp olive oil
- ¼ cup chopped parsley

Directions:

1. In a baking dish, combine the beets with the oil and the other Ingredients; toss to coat, introduce in the oven at 420 º F, and bake for 30 mins.
2. Divide between plates and serve.

Nutrition:

- Calories 156
- Fat 11.8 g
- Carbs 11.5 g
- Protein 3.8 g

Sage Carrots

Prep Time: 10 mins

Servings: 4

Ingredients:

- 2 tsps. sweet paprika
- 1 tbsp chopped sage
- 2 tbsp olive oil
- 1 lb. peeled and roughly cubed carrots
- ¼ tsp. black pepper
- 1 chopped red onion

Directions:

1. In a baking pan, combine the carrots with the oil and the other Ingredients; toss and bake at 380 º F for 30 mins.
2. Divide between plates and serve.

Nutrition:

- Calories 200
- Fat 8.7 g
- Carbs 7.9 g
- Protein 4 g

Dates and Cabbage Sauté

Prep Time: 5 mins

Servings: 4

Ingredients:

- 2 tbsp olive oil
- 2 tbsp lemon juice
- 1 lb. shredded red cabbage
- Black pepper
- 8 pitted and sliced dates
- 2 tbsp chopped chives
- ¼ cup low-sodium veggie stock

Directions:

- Heat up a pan with the oil over medium heat, add the cabbage and the dates, toss and cook for 4 mins.
- Add the stock and the other Ingredients; toss, cook over medium heat for 11 mins more, divide between plates and serve.

Nutrition:

- Calories 280
- Fat 8.1 g
- Carbs 8.7 g
- Protein 6.3 g

Baked Squash Mix

Prep Time: 10 mins

Servings: 4

Ingredients:

- 2 tsps. chopped cilantro
- 2 lbs. peeled and sliced butternut squash
- ¼ tsp. black pepper
- 1 tsp. garlic powder
- 2 tbsp olive oil
- 1 tsp. chili powder
- 1 tbsp lemon juice

Directions:

In a roasting pan, combine the squash with the oil and the other Ingredients; toss gently, bake in the oven at 400 º F for 45 mins, divide between plates and serve.

Nutrition:

- Calories 167
- Fat 7.4 g
- Carbs 27.5 g
- Protein 2.5 g

Garlic Mushrooms and Corn

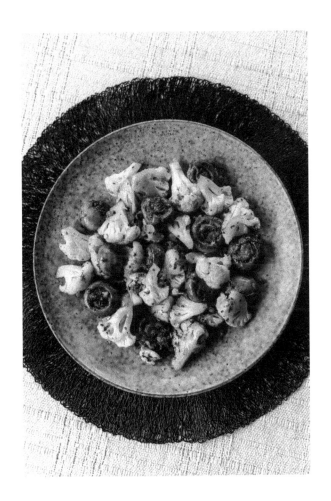

Prep Time: 10 mins

Servings: 4

Ingredients:

- 2 cup corn
- 1 lb. halved white mushrooms
- ¼ tsp. black pepper
- ½ tsp. chili powder
- 2 tbsp olive oil
- 1 cup no-salt-added, chopped and canned tomatoes
- 4 minced garlic cloves

Directions:

1. Heat up a pan with the oil over medium heat, add the mushrooms, garlic and the corn, stir and sauté for 10 mins.
2. Add the rest of the Ingredients; toss, cook over medium heat for 10 mins more, divide between plates and serve.

Nutrition:

- Calories 285
- Fat 13 g
- Carbs 14.6 g
- Protein 6.7 g

Cilantro Broccoli

Prep Time: 10 mins

Servings: 4

Ingredients:

- 2 tbsp chili sauce
- 2 tbsp olive oil
- 2 minced garlic cloves
- ¼ tsp. black pepper
- 1 lb. broccoli florets
- 2 tbsp chopped cilantro
- 1 tbsp lemon juice

Directions:

1. In a baking pan, combine the broccoli with the oil, garlic and the other Ingredients; toss a bit, introduce in the oven and bake at 400 º F for 30 mins.
2. Divide the mix between plates and serve.

Nutrition:

- Calories 103
- Fat 7.4 g
- Carbs 8.3 g
- Protein 3.4 g

Paprika Carrots

Prep Time: 10 mins

Servings: 4

Ingredients:

- 1 tbsp sweet paprika
- 1 tsp. lime juice
- 1 lb. trimmed baby carrots
- ¼ tsp. black pepper
- 3 tbsp olive oil
- 1 tsp. sesame seeds

Directions:

1. Arrange the carrots on a lined baking sheet, add the paprika and the other ingredients: except the sesame seeds, toss, introduce in the oven and bake at 400 º F for 30 mins.
2. Divide the carrots between plates, sprinkle sesame seeds on top and serve.

Nutrition:

- Calories 142
- Fat 11.3 g
- Carbs 11.4 g
- Protein 1.2 g

Mashed Cauliflower

Prep Time: 10 mins

Servings: 4

Ingredients:

- ½ cup coconut milk
- 1 tbsp chopped chives
- 2 lbs. cauliflower florets
- ¼ tsp. black pepper
- 1 tbsp chopped cilantro
- ½ cup low-fat sour cream

Directions:

1. Put the cauliflower in a pot, add water to cover, bring to a boil over medium heat, and cook for 25 mins and drain.
2. Mash the cauliflower, add the milk, black pepper and the cream, whisk well, divide between plates, sprinkle the rest of the ingredients: on top and serve.

Nutrition:

- Calories 188
- Fat 13.4 g
- Carbs 15 g
- Protein 6.1 g

Spinach Spread

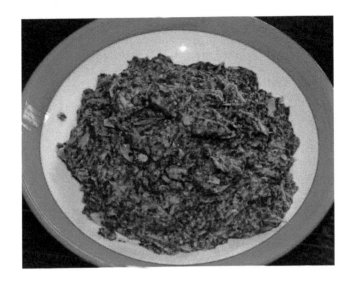

Prep Time: 10 mins

Servings: 4

Ingredients:

- 1 cup coconut cream
- 1 tbsp chopped dill
- 1 lb. chopped spinach
- ¼ tsp. black pepper
- 1 cup shredded low-fat mozzarella

Directions:

1. In a baking pan, combine the spinach with the cream and the other Ingredients; stir well, introduce in the oven and bake at 400 º F for 20 mins.
2. Divide into bowls and serve.

Nutrition:

- Calories 340
- Fat 33 g
- Carbs 4 g
- Protein 5 g

Mustard Greens Sauté

Prep Time: 10 mins

Servings: 4

Ingredients:

- 2 tbsp olive oil
- 2 chopped spring onions
- 6 cup mustard greens
- 2 tbsp sweet paprika
- Black pepper
- ½ cup coconut cream

Directions:

1. Heat up a pan with the oil over medium-high heat, add the onions, paprika and black pepper, stir and sauté for 3 mins.
2. Add the mustard greens and the other Ingredients; toss, cook for 9 mins more, divide between plates and serve.

Nutrition:

- Calories: 163
- Fat:14.8 g
- Carbs:8.3 g
- Protein: 3.6 g

Cauliflower with Breadcrumbs

Prep Time: 10 mins

Servings: 4

Ingredients:

- 2 cup cauliflower florets
- 4 slices of bread
- 1/8 tsp ground black pepper

Directions:

1. Place the bread in a toaster oven on very low heat. Toast as long as possible without burning (about 5 mins).

2. While bread toasts, trim leaves and stalks from cauliflower. Cut into individual florets.

3. Place 1 inch of water in a 4-quart pot with lid. Insert steamer basket, and place cauliflower in basket. Sprinkle with salt. Cover. Bring to a boil over high heat. Reduce heat to medium. Steam for 5–8 mins, until easily pierced with a sharp knife. Do not overcook.

4. While cauliflower steams, break toast into small pieces. Pulse toast in food processor until medium-sized crumbs form. Tip: If you don't have a food processor, break or crush the toasted bread into finer pieces or buy whole-wheat breadcrumbs and use 2 tbsp

5. When cauliflower is done, remove from heat. Melt margarine in another pan over medium heat. Add breadcrumbs and pepper. Cook and stir, about 5 mins. Add cauliflower to pan with breadcrumbs. Toss until well coated. Serve immediately.

Nutrition:

- Calories 45
- Fat 4 g
- Protein 2 g
- Carbs 5 g

Chayotes Stuffed with Cheese

Prep Time: 10 mins

Servings: 4

Ingredients:

- 6 small chayotes, cut in half, lengthwise
- 2 quarts water
- 1 cup low fat cheddar cheese, shredded
- 1/4 tsp salt
- 1 tbsp margarine
- 1/2 cup plain bread crumbs

Directions:

1. Wash chayotes and bring to a boil in water. Cover and boil at moderate heat for about 1 hour or until fork-tender.
2. Preheat oven to 350° F.
3. Drain chayotes, remove cores and fibrous part under cores. Scoop out pulp, being careful not to break shells. Place shells on cookie sheet.

4. Immediately mash pulp and mix with cheese, salt, and margarine.
5. Stuff shells with the mixture. Sprinkle with bread crumbs.
6. Bake for 30 mins.

Nutrition:

- Calories 129
- Fat 33 g
- Carbs 4 g
- Protein 5 g

Rotelle Pasta with Sun-Dried Tomato

Prep Time: 10 mins

Servings: 4

Cooking: 20 mins

Ingredients:

- 2 tbsp olive oil
- 1 cup sun-dried tomatocs
- 2 cup pasta
- 4 garlic cloves, mashed
- 1 cup vegetable broth

Directions:

1. Preheat olive oil in a skillet over medium heat.
2. Sauté garlic for 30 seconds. Then add tomatoes and broth.
3. Cover the mixture and then simmer for 10 mins.
4. Fill a pot with water and boil pasta in it for 10 mins until al dente.

5. Drain the pasta and keep it aside.
6. Add parsley and olives to the tomato mixture and mix well.
7. Serve the plate with tomato sauce and add 1 tsp parmesan cheese.

Nutrition:

- Calories 335
- Fat 4.4 g
- Carbs 31.2 g
- Fiber 2.7 g
- Protein 7.3 g

Garlic Steamed Squash

Prep Time: 5 mins

Servings: 4

Ingredients:

- 2 small zucchini
- Freshly ground black pepper
- All-purpose salt-free seasoning
- 2 medium yellow squash
- 6 peeled garlic cloves

Directions:

1. Trim the squash and zucchini and cut into 1-inch rounds.
2. Fill a steamer pot about 1 inch deep with water. Place pot over high heat and bring to a boil.
3. Place the veggies and garlic into the steamer basket. Place the steamer basket into the pot and cover tightly with lid. Steam for 10 mins.
4. Remove pot from heat and carefully remove lid. Pluck garlic cloves from pot and gently mash with a fork.

5. Transfer the steamed veggies to a serving bowl, add the mashed garlic and toss gently to coat. Season to taste with all-purpose salt-free seasoning and freshly ground black pepper. Serve immediately.

Nutrition:

- Calories 38
- Fat 0 g
- Carbs 8 g
- Protein 2 g

Grilled Asparagus

Prep Time: 5 mins

Servings: 6

Ingredients:

- ¼ tsp. garlic powder
- 1 tbsp olive oil
- 2 bunches trimmed asparagus
- 1 tsp. lemon zest

Directions:

1. Preheat the grill to 375 – 400°F.
2. Add the trimmed asparagus spears to a baking shcet.
3. Drizzle the asparagus with olive oil, garlic powder and salt, and using clean hands toss the asparagus well to coat with the seasoning.
4. Place the asparagus directly onto the grill grates and grill for 3-4 mins, until slightly caramelized.
5. Remove from the grill and season with the, fresh lemon zest, and serve.

Nutrition:

- Calories 45
- Fat 2 g
- Carbs 6 g
- Protein 3 g

Apple Glazed Sweet Potatoes

Prep Time: 10 mins

Servings: 4

Cooking: 25 mins

Ingredients:

- 2-1/2 cups unsweetened 100% apple juice
- 1/2 tsp ground cinnamon
- 2 lbs sweet potatoes (about 4 small potatoes), peeled and thinly sliced

Directions:

1. Combine apple juice, cinnamon, and salt in a large skillet. Add sliced sweet potatoes and bring to a boil over high heat.
2. Reduce heat slightly and simmer potatoes, stirring occasionally, for 20 to 25 mins or until potatoes are tender and juice has been reduced to a glaze. Serve while hot.

Nutrition:

- Calories 208
- Carbs 50 g
- Fiber 5 g
- Protein 3 g

Cauliflower and Potato Mash

Prep Time: 5 mins

Servings: 4

Ingredients:

- ½ tsp. flavored vinegar
- 1 minced garlic clove
- 2 lbs. Sliced potatoes
- 1 ½ cup water
- 8 oz. cauliflower florets

Directions:

1. Add water to your Instant Pot
2. Add potatoes and sprinkle cauliflower florets on top
3. Lock up the lid and cook on HIGH pressure for 5 mins
4. Release the pressure naturally over 10 mins
5. Sprinkle a bit of flavored vinegar and garlic
6. Mash and serve!

Nutrition:

- Calories 249
- Fat 0.6 g
- Carbs 55 g
- Protein 7.5 g

Mexican Cauliflower Rice

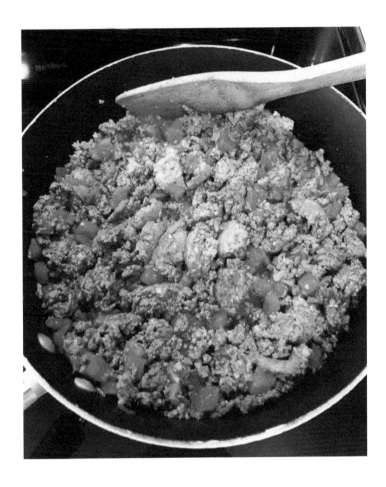

Prep Time: 5 mins

Servings: 4

Ingredients:

- 4 tbsp Tomato paste
- 1 ½ cup water
- 1 can fire roasted tomatoes
- 3 cup chopped onion
- 6 cup cooked brown rice
- 2 cup salsa
- 6 garlic cloves

Directions:

1. Add the listed ingredients: to your Instant Pot
2. Lock up the lid and cook on HIGH pressure for 5 mins
3. Release the pressure naturally
4. Stir in chopped cilantro and top up with your desired toppings

Nutrition:

- Calories 562
- Fat 25 g
- Carbs 63 g
- Protein 23 g